I0414090

The Essential Guide to
CBD & Cannabis Oil

By Max Burton

© Copyright 2017 by Max Burton - All rights reserved.

The following eBook is reproduced below with the goal of providing information that is as accurate and as reliable as possible. Regardless, purchasing this eBook can be seen as consent to the fact that both the publisher and the author of this book are in no way experts on the topics discussed within, and that any recommendations or suggestions made herein are for entertainment purposes only. Professionals should be consulted as needed before undertaking any of the action endorsed herein.

This declaration is deemed fair and valid by both the American Bar Association and the Committee of Publishers Association and is legally binding throughout the United States.

Furthermore, the transmission, duplication or reproduction of any of the following work, including precise information, will be considered an illegal act, irrespective whether it is done electronically or in print. The legality extends to creating a secondary or tertiary copy of the work or a recorded copy and is only allowed with express written consent of the Publisher. All additional rights are reserved.

The information in the following pages is broadly considered to be a truthful and accurate account of facts, and as such any inattention, use or misuse of the information in question by the reader will render any resulting actions solely under their purview. There are no scenarios in which the publisher or the original author of this work can be in any fashion deemed liable for any hardship or damages that may befall them after undertaking information described herein.

Additionally, the information found on the following pages is intended for informational purposes only and should thus be considered, universal. As befitting its nature, the information presented is without assurance regarding its continued validity or interim quality. Trademarks that mentioned are done without written consent and can in no way be considered an endorsement from the trademark holder.

Table of Contents

Introduction 1

Chapter 1: The Basics and Terminology of Cannabis Oil 3

Chapter 2: The Background and History of Cannabis Oil 11

Chapter 3: Major Phytocannabinoids 14

Chapter 4: Difference between Cannabis Oil and CBD Oil 19

Chapter 5: The Endocannabinoid System and Different Types of Endocannabinoids 24

Chapter 6: Health Benefits of Cannabis Oil 29

Chapter 7: Rick Simpson Oil 42

Chapter 8: Legality, Usage, and Preparation 45

Chapter 9: 10 Ways to Use this Oil 50

Conclusion 55

Introduction

Congratulations on downloading your personal copy of *The Essential Guide to CBD & Cannabis Oil*. Thank you for doing so. The following chapters will discuss some of the many ways that cannabis oil can be used in beneficial ways, along with details about its components, its history, and more.

What exactly are Cannabinoids?

Cannabinoids are compounds that occur naturally and are found in cannabis. Many different compounds exist in the plant including THC, Cannabidiol (also known as CBD), and more. In combination, these compounds make up the drawbacks and advantages of the medical marijuana field and all industrial products that are hemp-based.

Technically, CBD, along with all its sister compounds are phytocannabinoids, meaning compounds that come from plants. However, there are some other cannabinoid types you should be aware of.

For instance, our body produces cannabinoids, also called endoconnabinoids. There are also some that are created with chemical reactions (synthetic cannabinoids) in laboratories. We will discuss this in more detail later on in the book. As you will notice, every cannabinoid type has different effects on the body. Now that you are aware of the definition of a cannabinoid, how do these compounds impact your body?

The final chapter will explore 10 different usages for cannabis oil.

There are plenty of books on this subject on the market, thanks again for choosing this one! Every effort was made to ensure it is full of as much useful information as possible. Please enjoy!

Chapter 1: The Basics and Terminology of Cannabis Oil

More than 480 existing components can be found in the Sativa cannabis plant, and over 60 of these are called "cannabinoids," or chemicals that only exist within that plant. The best-known and studied of these chemicals, delta-9-tetrahydrocannabinol, is responsible for the "high" that some strains of cannabis cause. THC's effects are thought to be controlled and influenced by other components in the plant itself, especially the cannabinoids.

Subclasses of Cannabinoids:

Each cannabinoid can be separated into a different subclass. There are many, many different types, but for this section, we will focus on the most common and prevalent ones. Here are some examples:

-(**THC**) Tetrahydrocannabinols
-(**CBQ**) Cannabigerols
-(**CBN**) Cannabinol
-(**CBC**) Cannabichromenes
-(**CBDL**) Cannabinodiol
-(**CBD**) Cannabidiols
-(**CBT**) Cannabitriol
-(**CBE**) Cannabielsoin
-(**CBL**) Cannabicyclol

How do Cannabinoids Work?

Similar to opiates (substances like heroin, that come from poppy), cannabinoids impact the person using them by affecting certain receptors within the CNS (central nervous system). At the present date, two different types of these receptors have been discovered, and they are called CB1 and CB2.

The specific impact these cannabinoids have on the brain stand for the parts of the human brain they are interacting with. These interactions usually happen in the body's limbic system (the area in the brain that affects cognition, memory, and more). These interactions are distributed in parts of the brain associated with pain perception, as well.

Cannabinoids and their Differences:
The main distinctions between each cannabinoid is determined by how psychologically active they are. There are three classes of them (CBD, CBC, and CBG) have not been seen to have this type of effect. CBDL, CBN, and THC, on the other hand, have been shown to have psychological impacts in various degrees of strength.

CBD, the Most Prevalent Compound:
CBD is likely the cannabinoid that is most prevalent and contributes to about 40 percent of resin from cannabis. Interestingly, the compound might have effects that fight anxiety and also lessen the THC's psychoactive impacts.

In other words, a plant that has a higher amount of CBD might actually lessen the impacts of the compound THC, which will lower the plant's potency overall. Using cannabis that has less CBD has a heightened psychological effect with less unwanted side effects like anxiety.

Cannabidiol is one of the many natural chemicals that exists in the cannabis and is definitely one of the most fascinating and exciting cannabinoids. Also called CBD, this substance was once hardly heard of, and is now becoming a possible breakthrough treatment and nutritional component. This book will be about CBD oil, which is made from this compound.

Where is CBD Found?

CBD (cannabidiol) can be found in the flowers, stalk, and seeds of the cannabis plant, along with marijuana and hemp. Unlike a lot of the countless cannabinoids that we know about, this substance naturally occurs in large amounts within the cannabis plant and is easy to extract for that reason. Research has proven that CBD isn't psychoactive in the way that THC is. In addition, it's been proven to have many neuroprotective and antioxidant properties.

How it's Produced:

Cannabidiol can be made in two different ways. There's the natural method that occurs in wild cannabis, which is found in marijuana and hemp varieties of the plant. We will discuss this in more detail later, but the main difference between marijuana and hemp is the THC amount found in the plant. Marijuana is produced specifically for its THC, typically to be used in a recreational way, but hemp has only tiny amounts of the substance.

CBD, on the other hand, is naturally found in hemp and is not illegal in the U.S. the way other hemp products are. CBD that comes from marijuana is not legal federally, but state legislation varies from place to place and is currently developing. CBD is also synthetically produced in labs, but synthetically made CBD is regulated and illegal to possess unless you have special circumstances.

CBD Products:

As medical marijuana and its use grows, and legislation lags, countless people are searching for better ways to obtain cannabidiol, as well as more information about the substance. Since CBD naturally occurs in hemp, topical substances and supplements are growing in popularity. Cannabidiol (CBD) hemp oil items are and have been available for a few years, such as concentrated extracts, gums, drops, and daily supplements. In addition, CBD is used in skin creams, shampoos, and other beauty products due to its benefits in these areas (which we will also cover later on in the book).

Confusion about Marijuana and CBD:
There's no shortage of news headlines talking about marijuana and CBD, confusing them with each other and referring to them as "weed". This causes confusion and causes sensational, controversial headlines, especially when kids are given the substance. Cannabis is not the same as pot, or not in the way that a lot of people believe it is.

The Misunderstood Miracle Substance:
CBD oil is a very misunderstood substance. The majority of people out there are quite familiar with high levels of marijuana and the way it alters the mind. They may even be slightly aware of THC in the way that it makes the user high. What most people aren't aware of, however, is what else exists in cannabis and that not every strain of cannabis has a lot of THC.

What does it Help With?
CBD can be used to relieve arthritis, nausea, pain, and more. In

addition, it can help those who suffer from chronic illnesses. Although this does sound similar to THC, there's one major difference, and that is that CBD doesn't give you a high.

It Doesn't Involve Smoking:
A lot of people are hesitant or cautious about something that must be smoked to be used. Tobacco's ill effects are widely known and the majority of us wouldn't like smoking substances like marijuana, even without the high. However, CBD is able to be taken in many different ways and is not usually smoked. CBD oil, most often, is taken as it is orally, including gums, suppositories, and capsules.

CBD Oil and Pot Legalization Efforts:
CBD oil comes up a lot in legislation involving medical marijuana, but there are some legal experts who claim that the substance cannot even be illegal in the first place. The DEA has already lost numerous court wars because it cannot regulate items created from hemp and has no justification for trying to do so.

Since CBD has been made a part of legislation around medical marijuana, discoveries about hemp are being ignored. Due to the confusion between hemp and marijuana, a lot of those who benefit from CBD oil aren't aware of their rights about it.

Terms and Conditions Related to Cannabidiol:
We already explained that plenty of confusing words and terms exist in relation to Cannabidiol, so here is a list of some of the most important definitions in regard to the substance.

Cannabis: Cannabis is a flowering plant with three very different varieties; these are Cannabis Sativa, Cannabis Indica, and Cannabis Ruderalis. This plant has a large range of medical and industrial uses and applications and has been used medically, for oils and for its sturdy fibers for ages and ages. But Cannabis has also been used recreationally, as a drug, which has made it restricted in many places.

Cannabinoids: This is a highly diverse family of chemicals that has artificially created and natural substances included in it. Various cannabinoids have various effects and some have relaxing, soothing properties, while other types are considered illegal drugs.

CBD: This is a cannabinoid that is naturally occurring and is the second most highly prevalent component of Cannabis. It's safe to take and legal, but is still in THC's shadow regardless of its many benefits.

Hemp: Hemp is the varieties of the cannabis plant that are high grown and cultivated specifically for its seeds, oil, and fiber. These properties then get refined into products like hemp oil, fuel, rope, paper, pulp, cloth, resin, and wax.

Hemp Oil: This substance is obtained when benefit-rich hemp seeds are pressed, and it's a bit different than cannabis oil even though both of them are a product of Cannabis Sativa.

Psychoactive: This word refers to all chemical substances that are able to enter your brain via your bloodstream and impact your CNS (central nervous system). Some are psychiatric drugs, while others are dangerous, used recreationally, and can lead to addiction and other harmful side effects.

THC: THC is the most prevalent constituent of cannabis and has strong psychoactive effects. This is what causes smokers of marijuana to get high and as a result of this impact, the substance is regulated very strictly.

How is CBD Different?

In our modern world, countless supplements exist out there. But even though it's only recently popularized, CBD is known to be naturally soothing and calming. Scientists are also staying open-minded to possible wider uses of the substance later on. A lot of people are adding CBD products to their life for its relaxation benefits, but every person's situation is different and the only way to know whether the substance is right for you is to do plenty of research.

More on The Difference between THC and CBD:

Tetrahydrocannabinol (THC) and Cannabidiol (CBD) are the most prevalent cannabinoids present and naturally occurring in hemp. Considered phytocannabinoids (instead of cannabinoids or endocannabinoids which are artificially made), both THC and CBD mainly interact with certain brain cells, alone with cells in other body parts and organs.

Not the Same Substance:

Both THC and CBD are used in a wide range of ways and are comparable and similar on the level of molecules. Because of this, a lot of people have confused the two. Even scientists have confused the substances and believed that they were the same until recent times.

But the chemical functions and properties of these two substances are different enough for THC to be classified as a psychoactive drug while CBD is safe and legal all around the world. It's very important to know about the differences between these compounds so that if you use cannabis oil, you can seek out the right type for you. Realizing the differences between them will also help clear up confusion surrounding cannabis itself.

Rampant Misinformation:
Sadly, there's no shortage of misinformation about each of these substances. But this book is a great way to start learning about the differences, along with the benefits of CBD oil. Always do your research before deciding to use, make, or do anything else with cannabis oil. This guide will help you make the right decisions in that regard. What else is noteworthy about this amazing substance?

CBD Actually Works with Your Body, Not Against It:

As mentioned, CBD does work for many things, but you may be wondering how. CBD, fascinatingly, works along with your brain and body, rather than against it as many synthetic medications do. Humans evolved alongside this plant, so that could explain why our bodies handle it so well and why there are relatively few side effects when compared with other medications, such as synthetic opiates.

Chapter 2: The Background and History of Cannabis Oil

Cannabis grows naturally in nature and has been used for countless years by humans to soothe and fix a variety of health issues. The use of cord from hemp was discovered in a village site over 10,000 years old in Asia. Accounts differ about exactly when humans first started using it, but we can know for sure that we've been using it for a very, very long time.

The Introduction of Cannabis to the West World:

How did marijuana come from Asia over to the United States? In the opinion of the National Library of Medicine in the U.S., medicinal Cannabis use started at least a few thousand years ago and then was introduced to the Western medical field in the late 1840s, a surgeon who had discovered its medical benefits over in India. Due to its antispasmodic, anti-inflammatory, sedative, and analgesic properties, it was considered highly useful at the time.

Historical Uses of Cannabis:

The discovery of hemp cultivation and usage during this period makes the plant among the oldest known crops of human agriculture. Later on, in 6,000 B.C.E., Cannabis oil and seeds were used in China for food purposes.

Biblical References to Cannabis Oil:
In 1450 B.C., the Bible mentions Cannabis oil being used as a

holy oil for anointing. In the Hebrew version of the Book of Exodus, a recipe was described that was confirmed by respected experts to be cannabis, mixed with other herbs and olive oil. Anointed ones from this time were covered in this mix.

It's also been suggested that the anointing oil recipe that God passed to Moses had Cannabis oil in it.

The Egyptians' Use of Medical Marijuana:
Egyptians were discovered to have used the plant for medical treatments including inflammation, administering enemas, and soothing the eyes and uterus. Pollen from Cannabis was found in the tomb of Rameses II.

Modern Uses of Cannabis and Cannabis Oil:
Marijuana is used in modern day and California was the very first state in the United States to legalize medical marijuana. This was known as Proposition 215 and permitted patients to cultivate and possess marijuana to treat migraines, muscular spasticity, cancer, AIDS, and much more.

In addition, it's used in candles, soaps, perfumes, and even some types of food. It's a strong oil and you don't need much to get a powerful impact on your mind and body. The word cannabis (also referred to as marijuana) refers to the product from the Cannabis Sativa strain specifically grown for its sticky, potent glands, which have high levels of THC, which we discussed in the previous chapter.

The Therapeutic Value of Cannabis:

Worries about the harm of addiction and abuse to marijuana led to cannabinoids being banned for medicinal purposes in the U.S.A. and a lot of other nations back in the '30s and '40s. It wasn't until decades later that the therapeutic values of these compounds were recognized and even in our modern times, using them is very restricted for the average person.

Reducing Anxiety and Stress:

A lot of stress is bad for you, lowers your overall quality of life, and can steal years from you. For this reason, people with a lot stress are constantly seeking better ways to deal with their anxiety levels. Cannabis oil can relax the body, ease the mind, and release more pleasure hormones in the body, letting peace take you over.

The chemical compounds in cannabis, also known as cannabinoids, produce psychoactive or pharmacologic effects by activating specific mental receptors in the brain and body. This is especially prevalent in the immune system and nervous system.

The Origins of Cannabis:

Cannabis is originally from Central Asia but is grown all over the world today. In America, it's considered a classified, Schedule 1 drug, meaning it has a high potential for people to abuse it. This plant creates resin-filled psychoactive substances known as cannabinoids.

Most scientists in modern day agree that regardless of the mild potential of addiction to cannabis, cannabinoids' therapeutic value should be put to use instead of pushed aside.

Chapter 3: Major Phytocannabinoids

As mentioned before, the word "cannabinoid" can mean any of the various chemicals in Cannabis. Any time you ingest or smoke marijuana, these are what are causing the medical benefits produced.

The Main Cannabis Cannabinoids:

THC:

As many people already know, THC is the main compound responsible for the psychoactive effects of marijuana. This is what causes the high that marijuana is known for. THC offers a wide range of medical benefits, including (but not limited to) the following issues:

- Multiple Sclerosis
- Neuropathic Pain
- Alzheimer's
- PTSD
- Cancer
- Parkinson's Disease

CBD:

CBD, which stands for cannabidiol, is not as well-known as THC, but is just as relevant. Similar to THC, CBD's medical benefits continue to grow and grow. As mentioned before, CBD does not have psychoactive effects. As soon as the mainstream news discovered the medicinal benefits of CBD, a bunch of research came out to back it up. Here are some conditions that are treatable with CBD:

- Diabetes
- Psychotic Disorders
- Anxiety
- Depression
- Cancer
- Epilepsy
- Chronic Pain

THS vs. CBD, What is the Scientific Background?

In general, it's accepted and known that CBD is the safer out of these two substances (THC and CBD). Many studies have proven risks involved in long term THC-use, including psychosis and schizophrenia. It's important to note that when it comes to scientific research, correlation is not always causation, so THC may be connected with these disorders without causing them.

As we've mentioned before, CBD has more uses than THC, or at least that's what is believed at the time. CBD hasn't been studied as much as THC, so scientists believe that CBD has many more applications that we don't know about yet. In addition, the applications of THC have mostly been explored as much as they can due to medical marijuana research in recent years.

The Cannabinoids that Aren't as Well-Known:

CBG:

CBG stands for cannabigerol, which is present in the plant early in its cycle of growth. This makes the cannabinoid hard to find in more than small quantities. This cannabinoid is not psychoactive and can therefore be cultivated through hemp. Due to its medical potential, CBG is a big research target for the medical field right now.

In the year 1998, scientists in Korea discovered that CBG helped to slow down cancerous cell growth taking place in the mouth. Later on, it was shown to help against tumor effects of cancer cells in the prostate.

CBC:

Also called Cannabichromene, this cannabinoid comes in third place for the most common chemical found in marijuana as a whole. In certain marijuana strains, CBC takes dominance over the usually more common cannabinoid, CBD. This chemical is also non-psychoactive. Here's what it can do:

- **Anti-Tumor:** When CBC is paired with THC and some other chemical compounds in marijuana, it may be able to fight against breast cancer. Alone, CBC doesn't have as exciting or promising of tumor-fighting effects as THC, CBD, or CBG, but they work together to create a powerful fight against tumors.

- **Anti-Depressant:** In the world of science and research, there is actually a proven way to show whether or not a rodent is feeling depressed. When the mouse is held up, if it struggles to escape, it has an elevated mood. If not, it doesn't. CBC was proven to elevate the moods of the mice being tested.

- **Anti-Inflammatory:** CBC is helpful for treating inflammation by itself, but in 2010, it was discovered that when it's combined with the compound THC, it works even better. This discovery suggests that cannabinoids work well when used in combination.

- **Helps Your Brain Grow:** Research done in 2013 showed that CBC might help regrow brain cells. Despite how old you are, certain brain cells continue growing with neurogenesis. The affected areas work for learning and memory. Once these cells stop growing, risks for diseases such as Alzheimer's increase.

CBN:

CBN stands for Cannabinol, which comes out as soon as the dried plant flower has started going stale. When marijuana gets left sitting out for a while, CBN will multiple in it. This cannabinoid has the following medical benefits:

- **Stimulating Appetite:** UK researchers discovered that CBN helped to stimulate rats' appetites when they did a study.

- **Pain-relieving Benefits:** Back in 2002, researchers in Sweden discovered that Cannabinol had powerful effects on relieving pain. THC and CBN both can help to fight pain because they relax blood vessels and release endorphins.

- **Treating Asthma:** Due to its powerful anti-inflammatory effects, CBN was proven to help stop asthma related to allergies in mice through boosting their immune systems.

- **Sedative Properties:** Out of each of the cannabinoids, CBN might be the strongest sedative. In some research, it was shown to be as powerful and effective as Valium.

- **Glaucoma Benefits:** In addition to THC, CBN has been found to help lower ocular pressure (which causes blindness for glaucoma sufferers). This points to marijuana positive benefits on blood pressure.

Chapter 4: Difference between Cannabis Oil and CBD Oil

Cannabis oil refers to oil made from the entire plant, while CBD oil is just the isolated cannabinoid CBD. CBD products should only be made with whole plant, organic cannabis since this gives the best medical benefits and safety. CBD products that have been made with industrial hemp have some issues that should be considered.

Less Cannabidiol:

Industrial hemp usually has less cannabidiol than cannabis strains that are rich in CBD, so a lot of industrial hemp is needed just for a tiny resulting amount of CBD. Due to this, the contamination risk is higher and the plant may draw in more soil toxins, reducing the overall quality.

A Lack of Secondary Cannabinoids:

CBD derived from hemp, along with CBD powder that has been refined, don't have the necessary extra cannabinoids and medical properties that cannabis oil has. The medical benefits of the substance are greatly enhanced when they interact with THC and CBD.

The Story of Charlotte Figi:

When she was only five, Charlotte Figi had already been enduring hundreds of intense serious seizures every week, for years. Her dad decided to find alternatives to the traditional medicine they had been pursuing, and came upon an online video that talked about CBD oil's treatment possibilities. Through the medical marijuana program in Colorado, her parents discovered a particular strain of CBD at a dispensary there. They purchased some of it and extracted the oil, with the help of friends. Low-THC, high-CBD cannabis is a great and effective medical treatment because of its high therapeutic value with low psychoactive effects.

Charlotte improved with her first dose of the oil and went down to just a single seizure each week. Then her parents met two brothers who owned a large dispensary in Colorado and worked with them to cultivate a consistent supply of CBD oil to continue to treat Charlotte. This was what started a specific strain called Charlotte's Web. A lot of other parents of children with similar ailments understandably wanted to get their hands on the same oil, but they encountered difficulties with that. Legal issues and confusion stand in the way of understanding what CBD oil is and how to obtain it.

Understanding the Differences:

Today, many people are finding out about the miracles of CBD and hoping for information on obtaining some. To help you understand this better this section will focus on the difference between hemp-based CBD oils, which we already discussed a bit earlier in the book, and marijuana-based CBD oils.

CBD Oil from Hemp:

CBD (Cannabidiol) is known for its relaxation properties. When it's isolated, the cannabinoid isn't psychoactive and has been shown to help treat seizures. This compound is present both in Cannabis Indica and Cannabis Sativa. CBD oil from hemp is made from Sativa, which results in an extremely tiny amount of THC, but some level of CBD. Federally, producing hemp industrially is legal, but licensure and laws vary by state.

CBD Hemp Oil Differences:

But not all CBD help oils are the same. There aren't many cannabis professionals or researchers out there who would dare to defy the wonders and efficacy of CBD.

- **Bad Manufacturing Dangers:** CBD is often a powerful, potent product that has incredible benefits medically. But the methods by which it's extracted, manufactured, formulated, concentrated, and administered can vary widely in quality. Some clients have become very sick from badly manufactured CBD oil and products, which have mysterious ingredients in them.

- **FDA Regulation:** CBD from hemp is FDA regulated and sold as supplements, but the FDA isn't authorized to test products for effectiveness or safety before they're sold. This norm is way worse than most recreational and medical marijuana markets, which hold themselves to stringent testing and production guidelines, typically. Those guidelines usually exclude CBD that has been derived through hemp.

Medical Marijuana Manufacturers and CBD:

The brothers who created the Charlotte's Web CBD oil manufacture it under the title CW Hemp. Since the products have under .3 perfect of THC, U.S. federal law allows this to be shipped to your home. But many other medical marijuana manufacturers and producers are creating top quality CBD, as well. Charlotte's Web isn't the only option for high CBD product out there. In addition, there is Ringo's Gift, Sour Tsunami, Harlequin, and more.

- **Growing Marijuana Markets:** Since the mid-90s, several markets for medical marijuana have been growing in America (more specifically, the Western part of the country). States such as Oregon, Washington, and California have formed a way for seasoned growers to farm their medicines for patients. About twenty years later, those places, along with some new states, have expanded into recreational markets for cannabis.

  Cultivators in those markets create high CBD and high THC types of marijuana and mix them together into concentrates, topical applications, edibles, and more.

- **High Standards:** The markets mentioned above are known for holding themselves to stricter standards than typical agriculture for produce. In the present day, those who hold medical marijuana cards can get CBD items that have a lot higher amounts of CBD than the products that are hemp derived. Because of stringent standards and testing, it's also easier to find CBD products that are purer.

  When you are getting CBD items through the regulated the regulated marketplace, you should have access to the test results, ingredients, and origins of the product you're buying. Some labs may even give a full analysis of CBD content.

CBD Combinations:

CBD is most functional and effective when it's mixed with other types of cannabinoids. Cannabis has many different compounds, and about 80 of these are considered to be cannabinoids. As mentioned, THC and CBD are the main cannabinoids present in cannabis. They are both present in the highest amount and work very well together in a synergistic way.

- **Whole Plant Medicine:** Working with the entire spectrum of the occurring phytonutrients in cannabis is what whole plant medicine is all about. In the alternative and holistic medicine communities, this is a practice that is regarded very highly. This is very different from what most modern Westerners are familiar with in the medical field, which relies heavily on chemicals and pharmaceutical solutions.

- **Naturally Occurring Cannabis:** Before humans started to hybridize cannabis plants to concentrate more THC into them, naturally occurring cannabis probably had moderate amounts of both THC and CBD, in addition to other phytonutrients, CBN, CBG, and other flavonoids. Although it isn't approved for use of children due to its psychoactive effects, adding THC to therapeutic doses of CBD treatments adds a lot to the effects of CBD.

Medical marijuana cardholders in some states have access to CBD items and products that have various ratios of THC to CBD. This can be anything from 1:1 to 20:1, which offers a wide variety of therapeutic options. Hopefully this chapter helped you understand a bit about the differences between cannabis oil and CBD oil.

Chapter 5: The Endocannabinoid System and Different Types of Endocannabinoids

When you go over some of the scientific research around the medical and therapeutic benefits that cannabis and cannabinoids offers, you will quickly realize something. Cannabis has amazing impacts on our bodies. Just one herb with this many therapeutic compounds that appears to affect so much of our minds and bodies, how can that be?

The Treatment Potentials of Cannabis:

At many integrative medicine clinics, wide varieties of symptoms and diseases are treated with cannabis. This can mean Crohn's disease, cancer, eczema, Tourette's, insomnia, M.S., chronic pain, or epilepsy. This is only a few of the conditions that cannabis can help treat. Each of those conditions have varying symptoms, physiological effects, and causes. Patients may be young or old, while some are getting conventional therapy and others are seeking alternative treatments. But regardless of all these differences, many sufferers of these problems have discovered that cannabis helps.

The Cure-all Treatment?

Many doctors are wary when someone mentions a cure-all, panacea, or snake-oil remedy. Expensive solutions to health problems pop up all the time, with huge claims and hardly any evidence to prove their worth. But as the therapeutic benefits of cannabis are explored more, it's hard to find a lack of proof. Actually, new scientific research is constantly coming out about the medical benefits of this plant, even more than someone can find on more conventional treatment options.

The Need for Quality Information:

Within the past two decades, scientific studies published on the study of cannabis reached to nearly 9,000, and over 20,000 scientific journal studies were published on the subject of cannabinoids. This equals out to over two scientific articles each day in the past two decades. This shows a huge current scientific interest and investment financially in the study of this plant and its compounds. In addition, this also shows that the necessity for high quality study material so that good information is spread.

The Miracle Herb:

How is it possible for a single herb to aid with so many issues? How can cannabis give both curative and palliative actions and be so safe to consume while providing such powerful results? The will to answer each of these questions has brought scientists to discover a physiologic system that was previously unheard of, a foundational part of the healing and health of each human being and nearly all animals on earth. This is the endocannabinoid system.

The Endocannabinoid System Explained:

The endocannabinoid (endogenous cannabinoid) system was given this name in honor of the plant that helped it become discovered. This system is perhaps the most crucial of all in maintaining and establishing human health. Endocannabinoid and endocannabinoid receptors exist all throughout our bodies, in our immune cells, glands, connective tissues, brain, and other organs.

Maintaining a State of Balance:

In all of these tissues, our cannabinoid system is responsible for various tasks, but there is one main goal that remains the same, and this is the maintenance of a consistent environment regardless of external environment fluctuations. Cannabinoids help to promote homeostasis at all levels of life on a biological level, including the sub-cellular level, the entire organism, and maybe even the community and more.

Killing off Cancer Cells:

Autophagy is one example of the way the cannabinoid system helps to maintain the body's homeostasis. This is a process where a cell blocks of some of its parts to digest and recycle themselves. This process aids normal cells in staying alive, letting them keep balance between recycling products on a cellular level. However, it kills off harmful tumor cells by making them consume themselves. When cancer cells die off, overall homeostasis of the organism is enhanced.

Body System Interactions:

Cannabinoids and endocannabinoids can also be found where some of our bodies' systems intersect, letting coordination and communication happen between various types of cells. For instance, when an injury happens, cannabinoids stabilize the site of the injury to calm inflammation and pain. This requires three different action mechanisms on three types of cells for one specific reason; to minimize the damage and pain that the injury would cause.

The Mind and Body Bridge:

Our endocannabinoid system, due to all its complex purposes in our nervous system, immune system, and organs, is a bridge to cover the gap between the mind and body. When we seek to understand that system, we can understand the way states of mind lead to disease or health.

External Environment Influences:

Along with helping to regulate our cellular and internal homeostasis, cannabinoids also have a strong impact on our relationship with the outside world. On a social level, cannabinoids can alter our behavior, leading to sharing, creativity, and humor. As they mediate neuronal plasticity, neurogenesis, and learning, these properties can influence your ability to see the bigger picture, reformatting old and limiting patterns of thought. Knowing how to reshape these habits can help us stay healthy in a quickly changing world.

Cannabinoid Receptors Explained:

Tiny nematodes, sea squires, and other vertebrate organisms share this system as well, as a foundational life component of life and to adjust to changes in the environment. When you compare genetics of different species' cannabinoid receptors, scientists guess that this system has been around in primitive creatures since more than 600 million years back.

Gaps in Our Understanding:

Although it seems like we do know about cannabinoids, the thousands of scientific studies that have been published are only just beginning to bring light to the topic. There are probably many gaps in our understanding of how this works, along with the complexity of interactions within different cell types, cannabinoids, organisms, and systems. This will challenge scientists to consider health and physiology in completely new ways.

What We Do Know About Cannabinoid Receptors:

These receptors exist all throughout our bodies, are more numerous than other receptors, and are embedded into our cell membranes. When these cannabinoid receptors get stimulated, a few different physiologically effects occur. There have been two cannabinoid receptors identified by researchers so far. These are:

- **CB1:** This is predominantly occurring in our nervous system, organs, glands, gonads, and connective tissues.

- **CB2**: This is mostly found in our systems of immunity and structures associated with that function of the body.

A lot of tissues have both of these receptors in them and each are linked to varying actions. Studiers speculate that another, third receptor exists that we haven't discovered yet.

Chapter 6: Health Benefits of Cannabis Oil

Many different ailments and diseases, including metabolic syndrome issues, obesity, cancer, cardiovascular problems, osteoporosis, glaucoma, epilepsy, multiple sclerosis, inflammation, pain, and anorexia, are being helped or can be helped by the use of cannabinoids and cannabis oils.

What Does Cannabis Oil Help With?

As mentioned before, studies are still limited because of outdated laws and government guidelines, but a large number of patients are starting to wise up to the many uses and wonders of cannabinoid treatments. Let's look at some of the amazing medical benefits offered by this treatment choice.

Cannabis Oil for Treating and Preventing Cancer:

Cannabis oil can help cancer sufferers by killing off cancerous cells and also by reducing blood flow to harmful tumors. Research is limited and still being done, but this substance is thought of as an option for both preventing and treating cancer.

Can Cannabis Also Cause Health Problems?

We will get to the proven benefits of cannabis oil for treating cancer soon, but first we should address this common concern. When you think of someone smoking a joint with cannabis in it, there are obvious concerns about the risks involved in this, including lung cancer. In studies done on lab mice, the mice given strong doses of very pure THC appeared to have a decreased chance of getting cancer. In regards to cannabis possibly causing cancer (in the lungs by smoking), it's hard to say for sure since many marijuana smokers mix the substance with tobacco, which has been proven to cause cancer.

The solution to this concern is simple; using cannabis oil instead of smoking it. Cannabis oil does not have any known cancer risks whatsoever. With that in mind, let's look closely at some symptoms of cancer that can be treated with this wondrous oil.

Cancer Symptoms Cannabis Oil Can Treat:

Using this oil for cancer treatment or prevention can help to get rid of appetite loss, nausea problems, pain, weakness, and tumor size.

Types of Cancer it Can Help:

Several studies have linked cannabis with treatment of cancer such as melanoma, leukemia, brain cancer, breast cancer, prostate cancer, thyroid issues, lung cancer, colon cancer, and pituitary issues.

Killing Cancer Cells:

One study done in 2006 showed that CBD and THC significantly cut back the growth of cancerous cells in the breasts and reducing tumor growth.

Natural Alternative to Chemo:

Cannabis oil can also help cancer sufferers by inducing the death of the cancerous cells and providing a possible non-toxic option for a more natural chemotherapy alternative.

Help with Anxiety and Stress:

Anxiety, stress, and other related emotional issues seem to be on the rise, leading people to seek out natural alternatives. There are just too many side effects and worrying symptoms that come from long-term pharmaceutical solutions to these issues. Cannabis oil both stimulates pleasure hormones in our bodies and helps to relax an overstressed or worried mind. This combination can help to promote wellbeing and pave the way for a calmer outlook on life.

Processing Trauma:

Cannabinoids present in cannabis oil put these positive effects into motion within our body's nervous system. Some recent research has shown the tremendous potential value of this medicine in relieving stress and related issues such as trouble sleeping or even severe insomnia. One study done in 2013 showed that cannabinoids can help to treat the processing of traumatic life experiences and their related stress responses.

Promise for PTSD:

Studies showed that cannabinoids helped to minimize the brain's stress receptors and also that cannabis treatments can reduce the restlessness and anxiety related to PTSD. Whether taken orally or inhaled, cannabis oil can cause a large amount of positive effects in the nervous system, including increased feelings of calm and pleasure.

It can also help with the insomnia, anxiety, and other PTSD symptoms that come along with the disorder. Although more research needs to be done, the existing studies have shown great promise for the future of cannabis oil for anxiety, stress, and sleep disorder treatments. PTSD (or post-traumatic stress disorder) is a condition that happens after someone has suffered a life-threatening situation, such as a natural disaster, a serious accident, military combat, or witnessing trauma of some kind.

A study from 2015 showed that cannabis can effectively help military veterans in particular deal with their PTSD symptoms. The cannabinoids regulate and increase pleasure in the brain. Military vets who were previously in very bad shape from their PTSD were shown to improve with their coping abilities, anxiety levels, and insomnia issues. If cannabis can help someone who has suffered such severe trauma, what can it do for simpler forms of anxiety?

It Promotes Heart Health:

Cannabis oil has antioxidants in it that can help with heart health. Studies have been done on animals that show promise for strokes, heart attacks, and the treatment of atherosclerosis. One study published in Britain in 2014 showed that animal study results do show promise for human heart problems and that cannabinoids can dilate and relax blood vessels, helping to reduce blood pressure and improve the body's circulation.

Treating Asthma:

Asthma affects millions of people all over the world. It causes deaths every year and people have been seeking effective, natural treatments to solve this common respiratory issue. Cannabis is something that has been used historically to treat asthma in both Indian and traditional Chinese medicines. Cannabis oil can help for asthma due to its analgesic and anti-inflammatory properties and due to its ability to help open up the bronchial tubes and promote more air flow.

Obesity and Appetite Regulation:

It's no secret that cannabis can increase appetite and that it can help people increase weight gain or even recover from problems like anorexia. Cannabis oil is also effective for stimulating the digestive system, inducing hunger and helping people have more of an appetite. Cannabis oil can be helpful for stimulating appetite by releasing certain hormones that cause hunger, and hormones that cause hunger suppression may also be released with the help of cannabinoids.

Depending on the hormone being stimulated, cannabis oil can help to control obesity and reduce appetite. For this to work better, the cannabinoids need to be stimulated in the right way to stimulate the right, necessary hormones. Cannabis oil, basically, can effectively treat both eating disorders and obesity in the future. This is another wonder of the medicine, how versatile it is.

Antibiotic Properties:

Cannabigerol was tested for effectiveness on MSRA back in the year 2008. When it comes to antibiotic uses, CBG was found to be more effective than CBN and can be compared with CBD. In addition, CBG is anti-fungal and can kill off various fungi and bacteria.

Psoriasis Treatment potential:

Cannabis oil, especially the kind with a lot of CBG, can be great for skin issues. It can help lessen skin reddening but may also help with issues such as Psoriasis. In addition, CBG has been reported to relieve pain more effectively than THC. When you apply this oil to your face, it can help it glow and look fresher, shedding old dry skin cells. It also helps fix acne and solve dry skin issues.

Reducing Signs of Aging:

Oxidation and cell damage can speed up your skin's process of aging, causing wrinkles, lines, and dark spots. Due to its properties of high antioxidants, cannabis oil can help reduce this. In addition, consuming or inhaling marijuana can minimize anxiety and stress, which leads to rosacea, eczema, and acne.

Helps with Weight Loss:

Several studies have been done that show CBD's appetite suppressant impacts. These days, more research is emerging that shows a link between weight loss and THCV. In fact, a paper published recently showed that THCV can decrease body fat while boosting the energy and metabolism in tested lab mice.

Anticonvulsant:

THCV is another cannabinoid present in the cannabis plant that works well with THC. Some research states that this compound has 20 percent of the amount of psychoactive impact that THC has, but it may also mitigate some of the negative impacts of the compound. THCV has been shown to reduce seizures significantly in mice.

Neuroprotective:

If you've heard of smoking marijuana, you're probably aware that some feel slow after they smoke a strain with high levels of THC. But THCV can help to assuage some speech impairment and short-term memory issues that happen from this.

Help with Epilepsy:

CBDV stands for cannabidivarin, but hasn't been researched as much as some of the other cannabinoids. However, the small amount that has been done appears to be very promising. CBDV can be compared to CBD, but CBDV is a mildly degraded type of the same cannabinoid. This degradation alters the molecule's shape in a few small ways that are pretty significant, but there are still some benefits provided by the compound. It's an anti-epileptic, meaning that it can stop seizures in rats and mice.

Nausea-fighting Properties:

In addition, CBDV might be helpful for people suffering from gastrointestinal or stomach issues. Research done in 2013 showed that this compound is very effective against nausea.

Fighting Addiction to Cigarettes:

In one study, a group of smokers were randomly selected to receive a placebo or an inhaler with CBD in it. The participants were instructed to inhale each time they wanted to smoke a cigarette. Within a week, the participants with a placebo didn't see any change in how many cigarettes they smoked, while the CBD inhalers saw a 40 percent decrease in their smoking. The CBD inhaler lowered the amount of cigarettes they smoked without heightening their desire for nicotine. This suggests that CBD can help with the process of nicotine withdrawal.

Diabetes Treatment:

In one study with CBD, the advancement of the disease diabetes in healthy diabetic mice was reduced and prevented. There was no direct impact from CBD on the levels of glucose in the mice, but the CBD did prevent other harmful chemical production.

Fibromyalgia:

Fibromyalgia is commonly treated with anti-inflammatory medications, corticosteroids, and opiates. A study done in 2011 that looked at CBD treatment for the disease showed promising results for treatment. Half of the people studied saw a huge reduction in the pain and symptoms from their illness, but the other half, who didn't use CBD, saw hardly any improvement.

Mad Cow/Prion Disease:

CBD has been proven to cease prions, which causes Mad Cow disease. For the mice that were studied and had already been infected, CBD prolonged their lives by a week.

Our Endocannabinoid System and Health:

While the science of cannabinoids and cannabis continues to emerge, there is one very obvious and clear fact and that is that our health depends on a functioning cannabinoid system. From the moment we go through embryonic implantation, to growth and nursing, to healing from injuries, these compounds aid us in a hostile and changing environment.

Once this is realized, you may wonder whether someone can enhance their cannabinoid system with more cannabis, taken as a supplement. In addition to treating problems and curing illnesses and disease, is it possible for cannabis to aid us in preventing sicknesses, promoting health by aiding and stimulating the old system that we all have hardwired into us?

The Resistance to Herbal Healing:

A lot of physicians are resistant to the idea of recommending a plant to heal, especially when it comes to recommending smoking. The modern medical system prefers isolated, single substances that may be injected or swallowed. This model, unfortunately, limits our ability to discover cannabinoids' therapeutic potential. Unlike synthetic medications and treatments, herbal cannabis has many different cannabinoids, of which THC is one, that work together to create fewer side effects and better effects than just THC.

For Those Who Prefer Not Smoking:

Cannabis works pretty well when it's smoked and is generally considered safe, but many patients will prefer to stay away from irritating their lungs and will prefer other methods. These methods include topical salve, cannabis tincture, or a vaporizer. Patient testimonials and scientific inquiries both show that cannabis is superior medically to synthetically produced cannabinoids.

Returning to Nature:

Nature gives us everything we need to survive and thrive. Research into cannabinoids only proves this truth. Is it true that cannabis (used medically) may be the best remedy for curing a big variety of conditions and human diseases, a useful preventative measure for healthcare, and support for our carcinogenic and increasingly toxic surroundings? Yes, it is true. People in ancient Tibet, China, and India knew this, and Western science is finally catching up.

The Necessity for More Research:

Of course, as stated before a few times, more human-based scientific study is necessary to prove how effective cannabis can be. However, the proof is there and growing by the day, despite efforts by the DEA to discourage it.

Do most doctors know about how beneficial medical cannabis can be? Can they advise their patients about how to administer it, dosage, and other indications? Probably not. Even though two of the largest associations of physicians in the U.S. are requesting more research into the subject, a gigantic amount of publish studies, and a long history of therapeutic, safe use of cannabis, most modern doctors are still clueless about medical marijuana.

Times are Changing for Medical Cannabis:

Thankfully, this norm is starting to change because people are wising up and want inexpensive, natural, safe treatments that add to their life while working with the body, instead of against it. Medical cannabis fits the bill for this desire. This book is a great start for helping to spread the word about the use of cannabinoids, CBD oil, and medical marijuana in general.

A Case Report for Cannabis Cancer Treatment:

As stated, the scientific research on cannabis and cancer is still not very clear, but cannabis oil is still being thought of as a natural way to treat the illness. As mentioned before, it can reduce tumor size and get rid of weakness, appetite loss, pain, and nausea associated with cancer. The FDA hasn't approved this medicine as a way to treat medical conditions or cancer, but studies have shown that it possesses some properties that fight it, nonetheless. Here's a story that shows that.

A Failed Treatment Plan:

A study done in 2013 evaluated whether cannabis oil could benefit a teenage patient who had acute leukemia. For this person, a transplant of bone marrow, radiation therapy, and aggressive chemo were all given up on and treatment was considered a failure after more than two years of trying. The girl was very underweight and ill during this time. With no other solutions given by conventional medicine, her family started giving the girl cannabinoid extracts by mouth.

The Expectations for Her:

According to information in her case report, the girl was believed to have a terminal version of this disease. The plan was that no further intervention would be taken and that her treatment was done for. The girl was then put into home care and instructed to allow the disease to take her body over. It was believed that she was going to have a stroke within 60 days from that time.

Her Family's Research and Findings:

Once they received this horrible news, her family did some research and discovered that cannabinoids had been proven to inhibit tumor growth. Her family found that these substances are generally tolerated well by people and don't cause toxic side effects that chemotherapy does. They also found promise with a specific organization that had experience treating cancer using cannabis oil.

Getting Used to it:

To make the viscous nature and bitter taste of the hemp oil more bearable, they mixed it with honey (helpful for digestion) and gave it to their daughter every day. The goal was to increase the amount and frequency quickly to build the girl's tolerance up to the oil. At first, the girl experienced fatigue, increased appetite, and some episodes of panic while she was getting used to the new medicine.

Decreased Opiates:

Initially, the oil was given to her one time each day, but two weeks in, she was taking it three times each day. The results of this treatment were that she was able to decrease taking morphine, had increased symptoms of euphoria, experienced increased alertness, and disoriented memory. All of this is consistent with using cannabis. She continued using the oil for over two months. Her family would change strains on a regular basis as some were more helpful for alleviating pain and increasing appetite than other types.

The one who wrote this case report suggests that there needs to be more research done on cannabis oil since cannabinoids might show a selective approach when they attack cancerous cells, reducing the negative effects from agents of chemotherapy. Unfortunately, the girl in this story ended up passing away from a bowel perforation and gastrointestinal bleeding.

The Results:

This story shows that the advanced agents of chemotherapy couldn't control the counts of cells in the bone marrow and blood and led to devastating impacts and ultimately, death. The therapy of the cannabinoids, however, didn't have any toxic impacts or side effects. It only had psychosomatic results and even increased her vitality. It's also worth noting that using cannabis oil without psychoactive properties is possible by choosing other types of oil.

Chapter 7: Rick Simpson Oil

If you have read anything about medical marijuana, you have likely heard about Rick Simpson Oil in one form or another. This oil, which is also referred to as RSO, is a highly concentrated cannabis oil that has medical benefits. These benefits are especially apparent for those suffering from cancer. Where did Rick Simpson Oil come from originally, and who is the Rick Simpson behind it?

Rick Simpson's Story:

Rick Simpson came upon his fame with cannabis completely accidentally. Far before Rick Simpson Oil was heard or thought of, and before cannabis entered the mainstream as medical treatment, Rick Simpson was an ordinary man working as an engineer in Canada, back in 1997.

The Boiler Room:

He was working in the boiler room of a hospital and encountered poor ventilation and toxic fumes. This dangerous combination gave his nervous system a temporary shock, and he fell off a ladder, hitting his head on the way down. Rick was unconscious but when we came to, contacted his co-workers to let them know he needed the ER. Rick continued suffering dizziness and even ear ringing for quite some time after this event, but the medication he was taking seemed to have no effect on him, even worsening his symptoms, at times.

Finding out about Cannabis:

Once he watched a documentary on the subject of medical cannabis, Simpson asked his doctor about medical marijuana. Unfortunately, the doctor didn't even want to consider this as an option, so Rick took matters into his own hands and started sourcing his own. This led to a significant decrease in his tinnitus and an improvement in his other symptoms.

Rick Simpson and Cancer:

Just after the new millennium, Simpson noticed three bumps on his arm. His doctor thought that they appeared cancerous and tested them. They then discovered that Rick had skin cancer. Simpson had experienced success with treating his symptoms using cannabis before, and had heard that THC can kill off cancer cells in lab mice, leading him to choose to use it again. He treated the cancer on his arm topically, putting the cannabis oil onto a bandage, leaving it against the spots for a few days.

Believing in the Power of Medical Cannabis:

Once four days had passed, Rick took the bandages off and saw that his growths were gone. His doctor still refused to admit that cannabis was a suitable alternative to conventional treatment, but that didn't matter. Rick was a full-on believer in the miracle of cannabis oil. From this point on, Rick started to cultivate his very own strain, harvesting it to make a unique form of concentrate from the cannabis. This is how Rick Simpson Oil began.

Persecution and Perseverance:

Rick made it his goal and mission to distribute this oil to the people who were in need of it without charging anything. Rick helped to treat over 5,000 different patients with this oil, but the journey came along with its own set of unique struggles and setbacks.

His doctor not only refused to accept the benefits of cannabis oil and the profound impact it had on Rick, but he also got persecuted and arrested in his home country of Canada. His house was raided by law authorities multiple times and he lost thousands of plants to confiscation. However, Rick Simpson stick to his goal and continued giving out the oil. Even now, he is still spreading the word on cannabis oil and helping others. It's easy to see why this man is a hero in the medical marijuana community.

Chapter 8: Legality, Usage, and Preparation

People who utilize cannabis oil for treatment take it by putting it into liquid to hide the taste, or take it with a syringe orally. The frequency taken and dose needed varies on both the tolerance to cannabis and the patient's condition. The majority of patients will begin with a tiny amount, increasing their doses over time.

Seeking Reputable Sources:

It isn't possible to purchase cannabis oil locally or online unless you live in a state where that's legal. Some states will offer the use of cannabis to treat medical issues, but this might call for the necessity of proof of illness or injury, along with a note from your doctor. You may also consider joining a medical marijuana collective. This is a patient group who shares and grows their medical cannabis with the others in the group. If you do decide to use cannabis oil, it should always be bought through a trustworthy company that carries lab-tested and pure options.

Should You Worry About Interactions or Side Effects?

A lot of people are understandably concerned about interactions or side effects when starting to use cannabis oil for treatment.

Mixing Medications:

Cannabis oil can lead to a decrease in memory, concentration, or thinking and learning ability. For these reasons, the oil should never be mixed with other types of medication, including muscle relaxers, seizure medications, pain pills, anxiety medications, or antidepressants. Mixing these together could cause fatigue and drowsiness.

Pregnant or Nursing:

If you are already pregnant or planning to be soon, don't use cannabis or cannabis oil. Some evidence has come about that women using cannabis while pregnant or when their child was conceived may have increased the risk of low weight or birth defects in their child. In addition, cannabis should never be used if you are nursing.

Knowing Differences with Strains:

Many different strains exist for cannabis, and most of them are very different from each other. If you choose to use cannabis oil, as stated before, always ensure that it came from a lab-tested and reputable company that you can trust. Always go through safe, legal means of getting it so that you can ensure fewer side effects and the highest amount of benefits possible.

Making Your Own Rick Simpson Oil:

Making homemade Rick Simpson Oil isn't as hard as it may seem and involves a process that is similar to making your own cannabis butter or other types of infused oils at home. For the best results, Rick Simpson says that using Indica is preferred. However, depending on what you are trying to treat and your own unique condition, you may prefer to use something else.

Please note that the following recipe will result in a full 60 grams to be used for a three-month treatment program or regimen. For those who are seeking a smaller course of treatment, the recipe may be split up into smaller sections. For instance, a single ounce of cannabis will give you between three and four grams of the oil.

The Ingredients Needed:

- A pound of quality cannabis material.
- Solvent (2 gallons) such as 99 percent isopropyl alcohol.
- One 5-gallon bucket.
- A cheese cloth.
- A wooden spoon.
- One deep bowl.
- A rice cooker.
- One 60ml catheter tip syringe (plastic).

Follow these steps:

In order to make your Rick Simpson oil, follow these instructions exactly. Remember that you don't have to use Indica but that it is recommended.

1. Put the dried cannabis into the bucket, pouring your solvent over it until it's completely submerged.

2. Crush and stir the plant matter with the spoon as you add more solvent into the mix. Make sure you're using a wooden spoon, as stated.

3. Keep stirring this mixture for a few minutes as the THC from the plant gets dissolved into the liquid. At this point, about 80 percent of the compound THC will be dissolved

into your solvent liquid.

4. Use the cheesecloth to drain all of the liquid out of the plant matter, then put the plant matter back into your 5-gallon bucket to add more of the solvent liquid. Again, stir for a few minutes before draining the liquid from the plant matter, using the cheese cloth.

5. Throw away the plant material that is leftover, then transfer the liquid into a rice cooker, filling it up about ¾ of the way, then turning it on.

Although you don't have to have a rice cooker for this, if you aren't used to making cannabis oil, this tool will help a lot for keeping a steady, slow temperature. If the liquid gets too hot (over 300 F or 148 C), this will cause the cannabinoids to be lost because they will get cooked off. Don't use a slow cooker or crockpot since this can easily cause the mixture to overheat.

Keep this Temperature:

Your rice cooker needs to be kept at a steady heat between 210 F and 230 F, or 100 and 110 C). This will allow decarboxylation to happen. As your rice cooker gets hot, it will cause the solvent liquid to evaporate slowly. Keep adding this mixture into your rice cooker as you go along at a gradual pace.

Safety Considerations:

Please ensure that the rice cooker is kept in a well-ventilated, open area free from cigarettes, sparks, stovetops, or any fire at all. Solvent is a very combustible substance and can be dangerous in that case.

Your Mix is Done!

As soon as your solvent has completely evaporated, you can put the oil into a syringe to make dosing easier. The resulting oil is going to be very thick, so if dispensing it is hard, just put the syringe under hot water until it flows easier.

Chapter 9: 10 Ways to Use this Oil

Now that we have told you how to make your own cannabis oil at home, you can start using it. But in which ways can you do this?

Though THC is the main psychoactive component of the cannabis plant, there are also bioactive ingredients in the herb. One of these chemicals, cannabidiol, is believed to have powerful effects to heal disorders even without THC. Plenty of studies link cannabinoid compounds and cannabis oil to the treatment of health conditions and other diseases. Let's look at some ways that you can use this oil at home to improve your life.

Taking Small Doses:

The answer to the question above is yes. Studies show that small amounts of cannabinoids can help your body create more endocannabinoids, building up more receptors, as well. This would explain why some people who use cannabis for the first time don't notice a mental effect from it, but do the second time using it. This is because they needed time to build up more receptors.

A higher number of receptors heightens sensitivity to these compounds and smaller amounts tend to have a bigger impact. This creates an enhanced foundational level of activity in the endocannabinoid system. Small doses of this on a regular basis can help serve as a general health tonic and an aid for physical and mental healing.

Stimulate Your Digestion:

Taking cannabis oil internally can trigger hunger-promoting properties in your body. It's well-known that smoking cannabis increases the appetite, but even taking the essential oil is useful for inducing hunger. If you need to gain weight after an injury or illness, this is highly helpful.

Take it to Help Treat Stress:

Cannabinoid can be used to treat traumatic experiences and prevent impairment from stress. Many times, we believe that anxiety and stress is a part of life that we have to accept, with hard to balance social lives, families, and careers. But cannabis oils and their cannabinoids help to reduce stress, relax the mind, and cause peace and calm to the mind and body. You may find this helpful if you are undergoing a lot of stress in your life at the moment.

Get Rid of Pain:

Research has shown that medical cannabis helps to improve mood and pain levels in patients. If you're curious about how best to use this oil to treat pain, realize first that it's been used for a long time as an effective remedy. It can treat chronic pain and inflammation. Actually, many cancer and fibromyalgia patients going through chemo use cannabis oil for easing their symptoms and pain. A study done in 2010 suggested that cannabis can help neuropathic patients who just got surgery deal with their chronic pain.

Heal Your Eyes:

Cannabis oil may help prevent the degeneration of the eyes and also help to heal glaucoma. Glaucoma causes a loss of vision because of increased pressure in the eyes. Although cannabis can help to decrease this negative effect in glaucoma sufferers (and other people), the effects aren't permanent and only last a few hours. For this reason, it should only be thought of as a temporary solution. The patient would need to smoke cannabis every few hours in order to keep the effect going, which comes with a host of new side effects, like possible lung damage or cognitive impairment.

Improve your Skin:

Cannabinoids create lipids, which treat acne, dandruff, and dry skin issues. What benefits can be enjoyed when cannabis oil is used on your skin? It can help you shed your old, dead skin cells, adding to a healthier appearance for your body. This oil is believed to reduce free-radical damage and fight the stress caused by problems like acne, rosacea, and eczema. There have also been hair benefits found in cannabis oil.

Heal Heart Problems:

Cannabinoids can cause your blood vessels to widen and relax, which can reduce blood pressure and improve your circulation. Studies done on animals suggest that the cannabis plant can prevent heart attacks, coronary heart disease, hypertension, stroke, and atherosclerosis. There have been very limited human trials on cannabis for heart issues, but the research so far is promising.

Get Healthier Sleep Patterns:

It's been proven that THC can reduce interruptions in your sleep patterns and help you breathe easier at night. The cannabis oil has a calming effect which can reduce anxiety and restlessness in people who struggle with falling asleep. The cannabis's THC levels help insomniacs or others get to sleep easier. One study done by a Sleep Disorder Association found that THC is well-tolerated and safe for people who suffer from sleep apnea. THC was shown to improve breathing at night and reduce interruptions in rest.

What Else can it do?

THC can help cure nausea and vomiting in those suffering from cancer, and has been used this way since the '80s. In some cases, cannabis oil can help to relieve migraines and headaches. It may also help reduce the impact of schizophrenia, multiple sclerosis, and osteoporosis.

How is it Best Used?

After reading this book, you probably want to know the best ways to use cannabis oil. As stated before, it can be taken orally with a syringe or mixed into liquid to make the taste more pleasant. Always begin small and increase your dose as you go along.

Make Sure You're Following the Law:

Always make sure that you do plenty of research on the law where you live to ensure that you are staying within it and won't be punished. As we talked about earlier, legislation still has a long way to go, but it is progressing with time. As mentioned before, cannabis oil can cause some interactions or side effects, so always be safe!

Conclusion

Thanks again for downloading *The Essential Guide to CBD & Cannabis Oil*. It's my hope that you learned a lot about what this wonderful oil can do, its many medical uses, and some useful preparation guidelines. Marijuana has been used for thousands of years, in ancient medical practices, and to heal countless issues. Even though research is still limited and legislation prevents progress on this issue, this is changing as time goes on.

If you feel as though you can benefit from this oil, make sure you do plenty of research and then find a way to obtain it. If done right, this can help you a lot with your health issues. As always, make sure that you are following the law and keeping yourself safe from legal repercussions.

Cannabis oil can have some side effects, such as interfering with memory, concentration ability, and thinking or learning. You should never mix it with anything that causes drowsiness or fatigue such as pain pills or alcohol. Don't take it if you are trying to get pregnant or already are.

If you would like to learn more about CBD, check out my other book *CBD Hemp Oil: The Essential Guide to Cannabidiol*.

Finally, if you enjoyed this book, please take the time to leave it a positive review on Amazon.

Thank you and good luck!

www.ingramcontent.com/pod-product-compliance
Lightning Source LLC
Chambersburg PA
CBHW071125280526
45787CB00003B/1179